To Judy

May your baths
be full of bubbles
and suds

OX

Lisl and Laudt

SOAP

SOAP for body and soul

LISL AND LANDT DENNIS

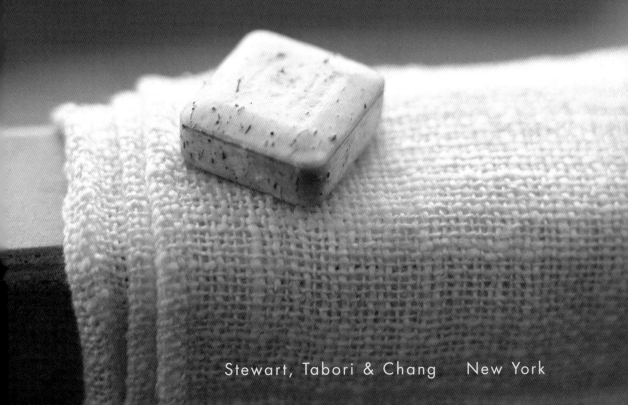

Stewart, Tabori & Chang   New York

Published by
Stewart, Tabori & Chang
A Company of La Martinière Groupe
115 West 18th Street
New York, NY 10011

Export Sales to all countries except Canada, France,
and French-speaking Switzerland:
Thames and Hudson Ltd.
181A High Holborn
London WC1V 7QX
England

Canadian Distribution:
Canadian Manda Group
One Atlantic Avenue, Suite 105
Toronto, Ontario M6K 3E7
Canada

Library of Congress Cataloging-in-Publication Data

Dennis, Lisl.
  Soap : for body and soul / Lisl and Landt Dennis.
      p. cm.
  ISBN 1-58479-135-7
  1. Soap. I. Dennis, Landt. II. Title.
  TP991 .D45 2002
  668'.12—dc21

                                                    2001057607

The text of this book was composed in Futura Book.
Printed in Singapore

10 9 8 7 6 5 4 3 2 1
First Printing

acknowledgments

Our gratitude for the help we have received in the research and the writing of this book is boundless. So many people have shared their knowledge and enthusiasm for soap with us, including soap companies, distributors, and stores. To all these unofficial co-workers we say 'thank you' many times over. The list also includes Wendy McEahern for her outstanding studio collaboration; Hugh Elliot, who worked miracles as a web searcher; Helen Pratt, our agent, for her unflagging pursuit of a publisher; and all the staff at Stewart, Tabori and Chang, including Sandy Gilbert, our editor, and Elaine Schiebel, editorial assistant, for their arduous devotion to the realization of the book. We also want to thank Nina Barnett whose thoughtful layout and design adds further dimension to the magic of soap.

contents

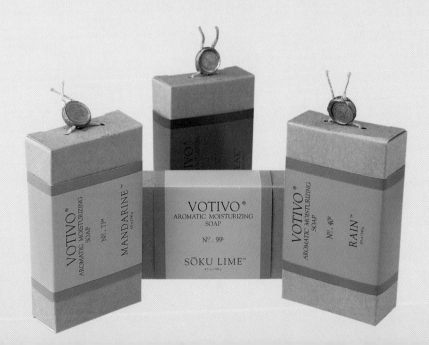

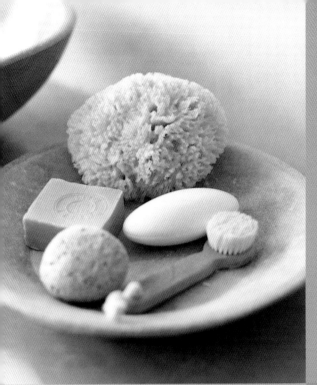

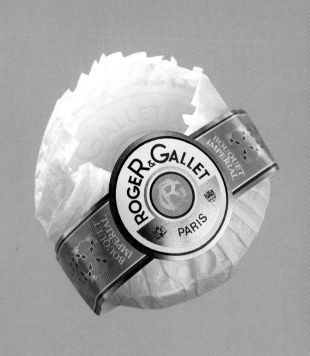

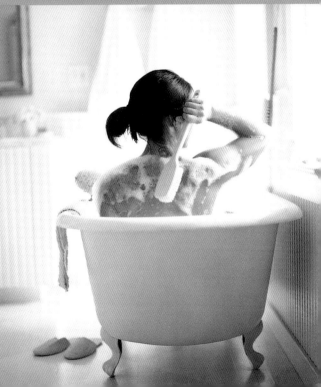

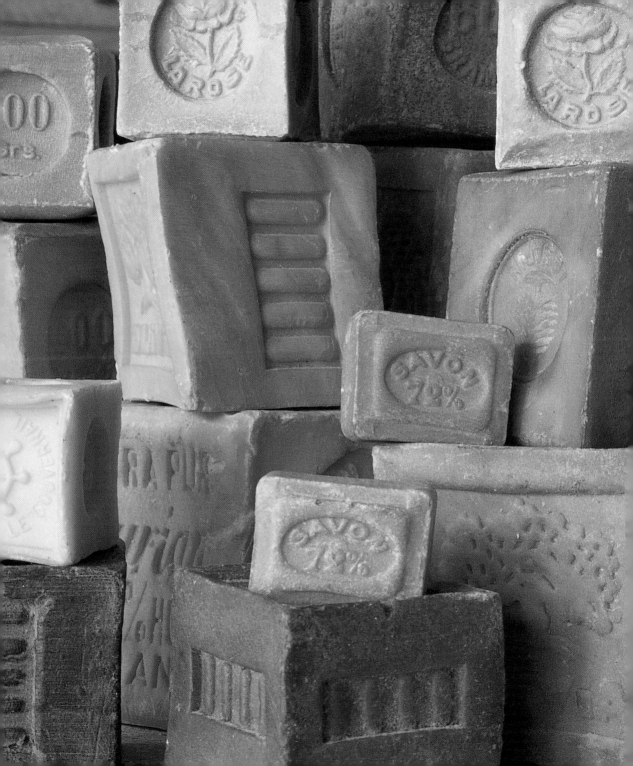

preface

My wife Lisl and I have been fascinated with specialty soap for sixteen years. Our interest began as we strolled through the markets in St. Rémy, Arles, and Carpentras in southern France. Allured by the high-quality peaches, artichokes, and leeks, our straw baskets became piled high with wonderful fruits and vegetables. And we always topped off our purchases with several bars of handmade soap sold by local producers whose booths were inevitably beside the flower stalls.

Who could resist the different soaps' exotic, sensual fragrances of lavender, wild thyme, honey, pistachio, and nasturtium; the soothing natural and pastel colors; the friendly, rustic French packaging? Provençal soaps became our passion. Our discovery of fine handmade soap on that trip has since turned into an addiction that spans the globe. Wherever we travel—Morocco, Italy, England, India, Japan, Bali, or throughout the United States—we are always on the lookout for specialty soap.

Many share our enthusiasm. "I came here just to buy pomegranate soap!" said one American woman we met in Florence. Her fervor brought her to the crowded counter of the seventeenth-century apothecary of Santa Maria Novella. "I love knowing I'm using a soap that was once used by Catherine dé Medici."

Many, like the American woman in Florence, have found their perfect soap. However, to most there is an overwhelming choice to be made from myriad soap products from all over the world. It is our hope that the information provided in this book on the wonderful varieties of soap, as well as the soap glossary and resource list, will guide every connoisseur through this seemingly indecipherable maze.

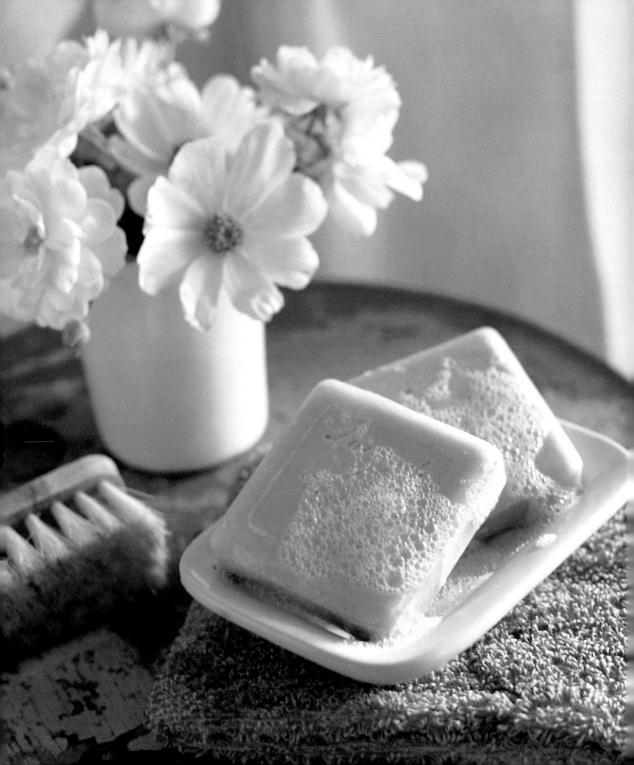

a brief history of soap

Bathing with soap is more than just a mundane daily ritual like taking vitamins or brushing one's teeth. Feeling clean is universally pleasurable, and for that reason, it is not surprising that soap has such an interesting history.

The earliest known depiction of a person bathing with a soaplike material can be found on clay cylinders from Babylon dating from about 2800 B.C. Later, in 1700 B.C., King Minos of Crete had a sophisticated plumbing system built in his palace at Knossos. Perhaps he spent as many enjoyable hours in his bathtub as Cleopatra did in her shallow bath more than 1,000 years later, where attendants poured water and essential oils over the fabled Egyptian queen. Whether she used a soap-like substance is not known.

Of course, one does not have to be royalty to enjoy the luxury of a soapy bath. In fact, Roman peasant women were the first to discover the base formula for "modern" soap sometime around 1000 B.C. The women noticed the clay from the banks of the Tiber—that was often embedded with sacrificial-animal tallow and ashes from the temple altars of Mount Sapo—assisted in cleaning their wash. By applying a little of the "sapo" clay, the laundresses had inadvertently discovered the chemical process of making soap, now termed saponification. Today, sapo continues to be the root word for soap in many modern languages. In Italian, it is sapone; in French, savon; in Turkish, sabun; in Spanish, jabon; in Dutch, septo; and in Hungarian, szappan.

The ethereal and temporal qualities of cleanliness are both praised and consecrated in the Old Testament. Moses sanctified the purifying agents praised later by the prophets Jeremiah and Malachi when he said—in so many words—to the Israelites, "To honor God in body and soul, take a bath."

Later, at the peak of ancient Rome's obsession with cleanliness, the city boasted eleven enormous and elaborate public baths, or thermae. Emperor Caracalla's thirty-acre water world, where operas are performed today, was Rome's largest. The city could also lay claim to more than 1,350 public fountains and cisterns.

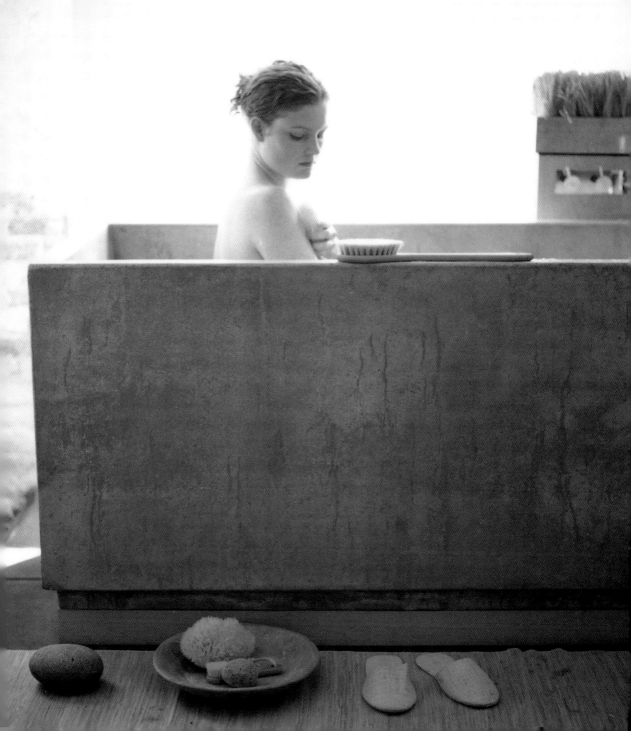

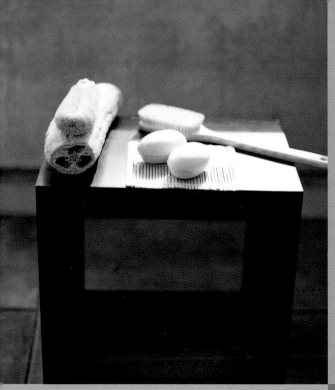

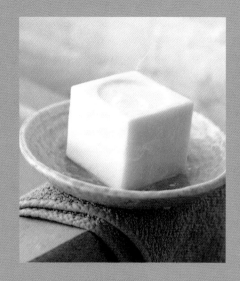

In Morocco, women wash themselves with *savon-beldi*, or "soap from the country." Made from olive oil, this soap is famed for its skin-softening quality.

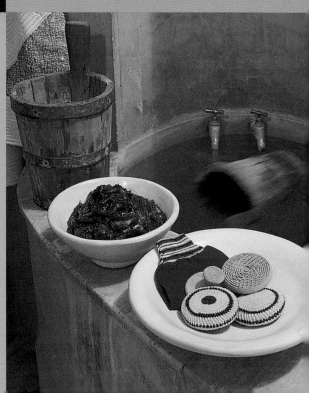

With thirteen aqueducts bringing water to Rome, citizens used about 300 gallons a day per capita—four times as much as today's average American family uses. An inscription engraved around 130 A.D. on the forum pavement of Thamugadi, reads, "*Venari, lavare, ludere, ridere, hoc est vivere*," "To hunt, to bathe, to play and to laugh, this is to live."

With the decline of the Roman Empire and the rise of Christianity, appalling filth spread throughout Europe. The clergy, shuddering at the debauchery and promiscuity that took place in Roman baths, condemned parishioners who bathed. In the following ten centuries, the faithful, from France to Jerusalem, further corrupted the denunciation into a belief that the holy sanctity of baptism could only be retained without bathing. "To those that are well, and especially the young, bathing should seldom be permitted," Saint Benedict decreed in the sixth century.

Throughout the Dark Ages, plagues swept the Continent, killing hundreds of thousands. Devastating epidemics of infectious diseases, rampant infant mortality, and short lifespans were all common during the period. Historians coined the era "the one thousand years of filth."

When European knights returned from their crusades in the Near East, however, they were full of praise for the delights of the *hammam*, a sensuous public or private bath, which continues to be popular in Islamic countries, especially Morocco. More than a place to bathe and be massaged, the *hammam* is a refuge where one goes to be restored, silent, and soulful. After centuries of repression, Europeans delighted in the renaissance of the bath, which included such extravagances as floating tables for eating and gaming. There were also large galleries for spectators to enjoy the view of the splashing bathers. Before long, monks and nuns alike began to have bathing facilities and to make their own soap.

France, Spain, and Italy during this period soon became leading centers of soap making in Europe. Olive oil became increasingly popular for soap manufacture instead of primitive animal tallow. The availability of locally milled olive oil made Mediterranean cities well known for their high-quality soap, especially Genoa, Italy and Marseilles, France. In Castilla, Spain, the area's great groves of olive trees were "harvested" by soap companies as well as farmers.

Marseilles, on the southern coast of France, was perhaps the most important of these soap-making centers. With a profusion of olive trees and saltwort (a source of soda) from the adjacent marshes of the Camargue, the city's citizens had the finest olive oil and soda ash at their disposal.

To ensure soap manufacturers utilized only these superior ingredients, in 1688 Louis XIV decreed the "Edict of Colbert." The law prohibited *Savon de Marseilles* (a general appellation and not the name of a brand) from containing animal fats, fragrance, and color. The soap had to contain 72 percent pure olive oil, in addition to copra and palm oils. The square, dun-colored cubes of *Savon de Marseilles* rapidly became the most popular soap in France and was used for both washing clothes and bodies. This legendary, all-natural soap continues to be esteemed today.

It took longer for Northern Europeans to become reacquainted with soap. The Celts are credited for reintroducing Britain to the delights of bathing. In 1399, Henry IV instituted the "Order of the Bath" whereby his nobles would bathe at least once in their lives as part of their dubbing. London and Coventry eventually became soap centers. The soaps they produced were made of rendered fat and imported oil.

The demand for soap soon became sufficient enough for soap guilds to spring up. Guilds quickly learned to keep careful watch over their soap recipes. They even began to brand their products. Early soaps were frequently embossed with spheres, the sun, half moons, or a lily.

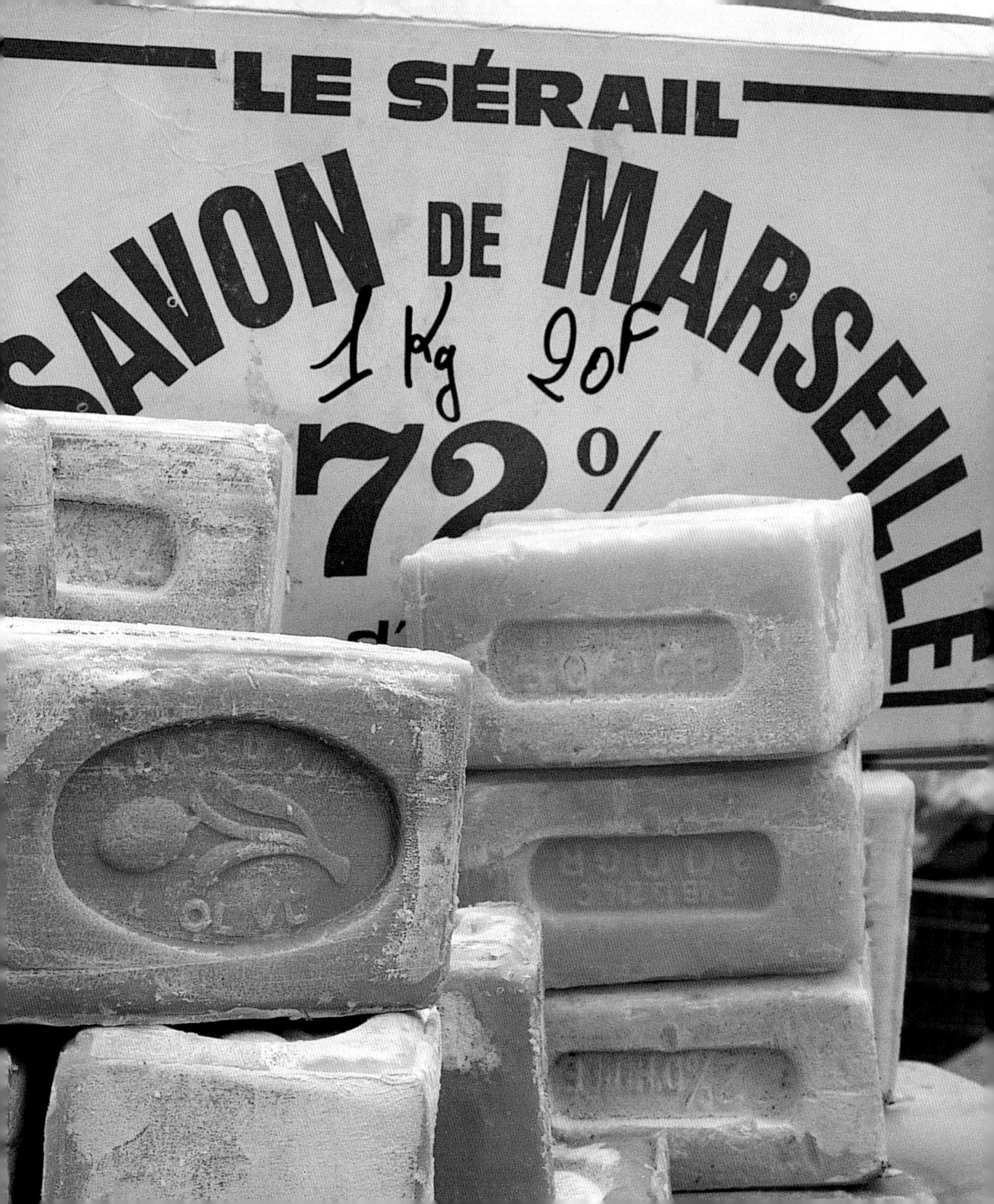
LE SÉRAIL
SAVON DE MARSEILLE
1 Kg 20F
72%

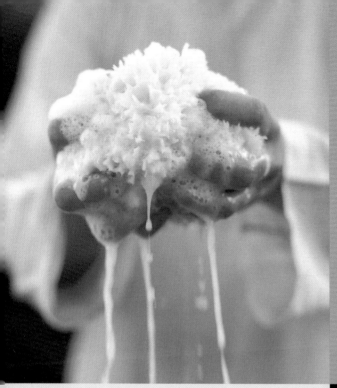

Once indoor bathrooms became the norm in the late nineteenth century rather than the exception, soap became a regular staple on the public's shopping list.

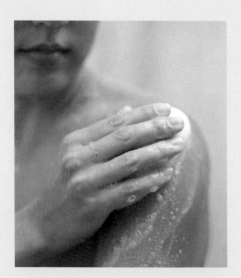

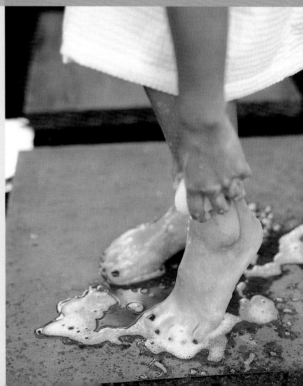

Soon, soap became so widespread that the crown took an interest. In one year alone, 1622, James I taxed soap makers the equivalent of $5 million in today's currency. In 1632 under Charles I, all soap pans were fitted with a padlock to prevent tax evaders. A tax inspector was required to be present in order to unlock them at every soap boiling.

After a while, soap became too expensive for most of the British population to afford. Unfortunately, science had not yet recognized the connection between hygiene and disease—a contributing factor to the 1665 plague that killed 75,000 people in London alone. Sadly, soap manufacturing continued to spiral downward as the soap tax levied rose to between 1 and 3 pence per pound, the latter being a staggering 100 percent tax of the total soap manufacturing cost.

Oliver Cromwell imposed even greater taxes in 1712, driving soap completely out of the reach of the lower classes. Ironically, as art and intellectual pursuits attained great heights, personal hygiene returned to a gagging low. Body odors were masked with heavy perfumes and dirt was covered, especially on the face, with a thick layering of powders and paints.

It was not until 1853 that Prime Minister Gladstone reluctantly repealed the last English soap tax. Shortly after the repeal, the British people could finally afford soap. The motto "Let the people be clean" symbolized a practical way to reduce disease, keep people working, and allow the economy to rise.

Around this time, William Lever was working in his father's grocery store in Bolton, England, where he cut slabs of soap and wrapped them in brown paper for customers. During slow periods, he read from his favorite book *Self Help*. Triggered by the quote, "A rut is like a grave, only longer," Lever urged his father to expand the operation by manufacturing soap. Lever Company, the family's soap business, was registered in 1884. The name "Sunlight" was printed on the Lever soaps, and breaking from tradition, each bar was individually wrapped in imitation parchment paper.

An immediate success, Sunlight paved the way for brand identification in the crowded soap market. With demand soaring, Lever planted seventeen acres of palm trees in the Congo for the production of palm oil. The oil was used in his expanded line, which grew to include Lux, Persil, and Lifebuoy.

With more than forty tons of his most popular soap sold in England by the mid-1890s, Lever was inspired to find new ways to increase his soap sales. The Lever Company published pamphlets on healthful hints, gave away puzzles, and organized widely publicized washing contests. Also savvy to catch on to the growing influence of advertising, Lever commissioned famous illustrators to design ads, which were displayed throughout England in railway stations and major streets.

Eventually evolving into the Unilever Company, one of today's largest global conglomerates, the firm's soap line continues to be popular worldwide. Among its many acquisitions is A. & F. Pears Ltd., producers of a translucent glycerine soap which was first manufactured in England in 1789 as an alternative to the highly alkaline soaps of the day. Clearly better than any other soap on the market, it had a certain cachet. Mr. Pears signed each wrapper personally in ink. Two other important British toiletry companies founded in the eighteenth century and still selling their soaps today are Yardley of London and Floris.

Soap's large-scale commercial explosion, outside of England, had begun in 1791 when the Frenchman Nicolas Leblanc patented a scientific breakthrough in the manufacture of soap. Leblanc invented a way to use common table salt to produce soda ash (sodium bicarbonate), the active ingredient in ashes that combines with fat to form soap.

Another major breakthrough in soap technology occurred in 1811. The French chemist Michel Eugene Chevreul discovered the chemical nature of fats and oil. Then in the mid-1800s, Belgian chemist Ernest Solvay took the manufacture of soap still further. He invented the ammonia process, a more efficient way to use salt to make soda ash. This reduced the price of soda and increased both the quality and quantity of soda available for soap manufacture.

As soap grew in popularity and became easy to obtain in Europe, it took on various incarnations: soap for bathing, soap for laundry, soap for household cleaning. Over the past two centuries, several European entrepeneurs have created noteworthy soaps with strong identities. In 1976, Anita Roddick founded The Body Shop in Brighton, England. A brilliant marketing executive, she recognized the vast market for toiletries that are handmade, naturally inspired, and promote an underlying commitment to animal and environmental protection.

Today, Roddick's products have more than 1,500 outlets in forty-seven countries. Mark Constantine, who at one time had a creative partnership with Roddick, has founded his own distinctive international chain, Lush. Harking back to the past, long soap loaves are cut into slices. Lush soaps have evocative names such as Angels on Bare Skin and Dream Cream.

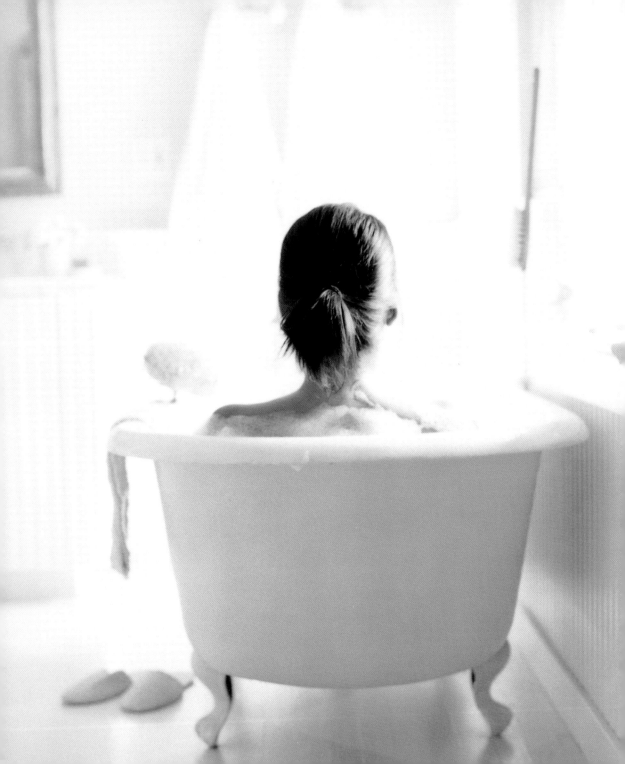

Soap emigrated to the Americas in the seventeenth century. What Europeans in the New World didn't know was that the Native Americans had already discovered a form of soap. For example, the Navajo created a soaplike solution by peeling, slicing, and pounding yucca root and mixing the resulting mush with water to make suds.

Settlers made sure to bring with them Old World methods and recipes for soap aboard the ships that brought them from England. Spurred on by John Wesley's famous imperative that "Cleanliness is, indeed, next to Godliness," hardworking colonists made soap in iron kettles in their own backyards. Fat drippings from the kitchen and wood ashes from the stove were carefully stored away to make the soap—normally an annual family affair that preceded spring cleaning. Soap peddlers, also known as soap boilers and tallow chandlers, went door-to-door, taking a month's accumulation of kitchen grease as part payment from housewives for a supply of ready-made soap and candles.

By 1795, there were soap manufacturers in all major towns along the eastern seaboard, and America was exporting ashes for English soap makers to use. With facilities for collecting ashes, called "ashies," throughout the nation, the United States exported more than $1 million of ash to England in the mid-1850s.

Eager to take advantage of the ever-growing trend in hygiene, Benjamin Franklin introduced the first bathtub to America. It was a copper model of the French *sabot*, with a small oven in the back to heat the water. It was called a "slipper bath" because the bather was submerged in water the whole length of the body. Later a drain was put at one end of the tub, making bathing truly sanitary.

In 1851, when President Millard Fillmore had the first bathtub installed in the White House, the nation knew that personal cleanliness had reached a level of utmost importance. In 1872, Thomas Crapper, a plumbing genius, unveiled a flushing water closet. After that, every home aspired to have a bathroom in which there would be a toilet, a tub, eventually a shower, hot and cold running water, and a supply of bath soap.

In the United States, pharmacies in the eighteenth and nineteenth centuries were frequently soap makers. Caswell-Massey, founded in 1752 in Newport, Rhode Island, is a good example. Still in business today and relocated to New York City, the company gained a great deal of attention when it began to use whale oil in its soaps in the 1860s. Today, these soaps are no longer in the company catalogue, but Caswell-Massey's Number Six, a favorite of George Washington, is still available.

Colgate & Company's Cashmere Bouquet is one of the oldest American specialty soaps still on the American market. Offered to the public for the first time in 1872, each hand-wrapped bar was either white with mottled brown resin (which had been added as filler) or pure white, a finer, more expensive product.

A generation later Samuel Colgate was inspired to import French perfumes to put in the company's product. He expanded the company's line to more than 100 different kinds of soaps. Popular as a sachet for women to put in drawers where their linens, lingerie, and handkerchiefs were kept, Cashmere Bouquet sold for an exorbitant twenty-five cents. Despite the high price for the time, by 1883 the soap was outselling all European soaps.

The Industrial Revolution, coupled with sweeping housing improvements, sent soap sales skyrocketing from 1890 to 1920. In the increasingly industrialized United States, factory soap companies began to replace artisanal soap makers. Automatic soap presses were introduced in 1912 and wrapping machines in 1914. With more efficient production, along with greater quality control, soap could be made

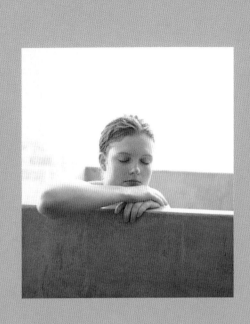

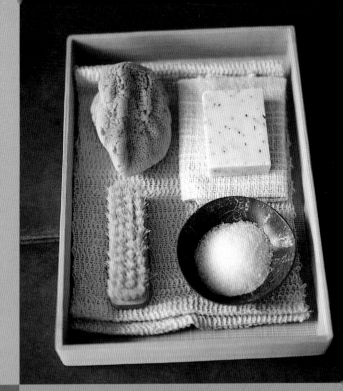

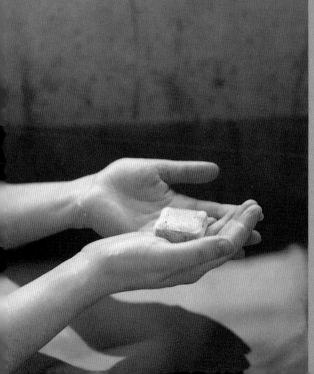

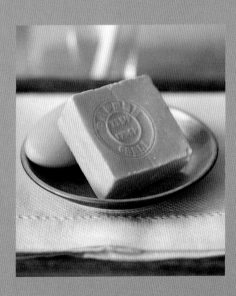

continuously in large quantities. The warm soap was whipped and extruded, then cut and/or stamped into the formed bars we recognize today.

At this time production costs for soap manufacturing dropped dramatically. With retail prices for soap falling, the public went on a soap-buying spree. William Procter, a soaper, and James Gamble, a candlemaker, were there to meet the demand. Capitalizing on the fact that Procter & Gamble's products, which included soap and candles, were relatively inexpensive, quickly consumed, and were in demand, the two men saw their company grow. However, nothing would prepare them for the amazing success that an assembly line worker stumbled onto in 1879. Leaving a soap mixer on during lunch hour, the employee returned to find that the batch of soap was lighter than normal because of the extra air that had been whipped into it. Vetoing the employee's wish to reboil the soap, management thought they had something in the accidental lightness. The white soap, as it was then called, was shipped out for sale and became an instant hit. Inspired by Psalm 45, Verse 8—"All thy garments smell of myrrh, and aloes, and cassia, out of the ivory palace, whereby they have made thee glad"—Procter renamed the soap "Ivory."

Turning into a multibillion dollar company producing hundreds of household products, Procter & Gamble was not without competition. During the 1900s, other American brands, often produced by the same companies, have made a name for themselves, too, including Camay, Dial, Dove, Safeguard, and Shield.

As competition increased, the need to develop customer loyalty became important. Soap manufacturers sought ways to distinguish themselves through the catchy brand names for their products, including Telephone Soap to commemorate the gadget invented by Alexander Graham Bell. Manufacturers also began to advertise. And companies sought endorsements for their products from leading glamour girls of the time, including Lillie Langtry, Lillian Russell, and Adelina Patti.

Procter & Gamble was the first company to take to the airwaves to advertise its product. And others followed suit. Soap companies became the major sponsors of "soap operas," and early radio listeners unwittingly became product conscious as they turned their dials to *The Tale of Mrs. Reilly, The Guiding Light, The Edge of Night, Search for Tomorrow,* or the popular *Ma Perkins.*

Towards the end of the twentieth century, the number of specialty soaps and their volume of sales rose. Neutrogena is said to be the most popular specialty soap in the United States today. A mild, clear soap with the company name, Neutrogena leaves essentially no residue. This Los Angeles-based company's specialized soap products appeal to today's health and beauty conscious consumer. In fact, the market for specialty soap in the United States and throughout the world has become huge. No one is impervious to the allure of a good bar of soap.

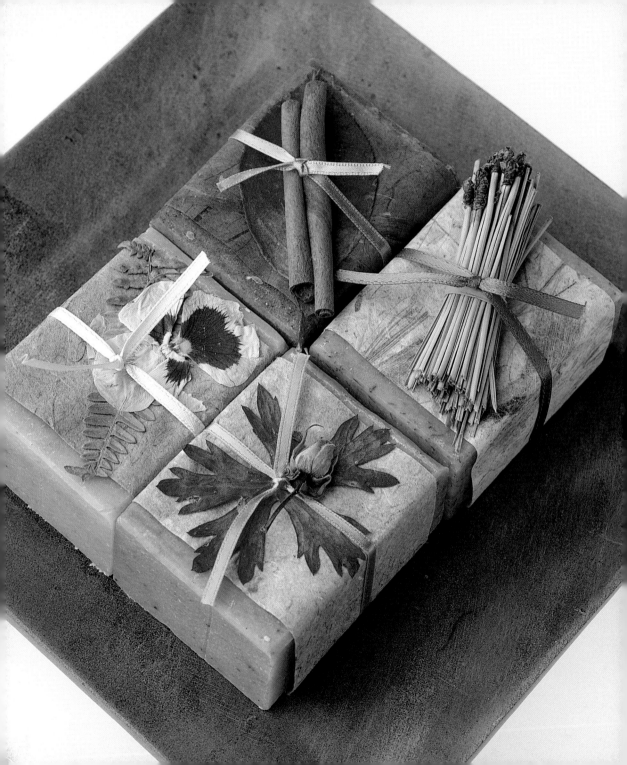

current trends in soap

Today's soap buyer is less influenced by mass-marketed, heavily advertised campaigns. "Niche marketing" is a major reason for the boom in current specialty soap sales. Luxury brands of exotic soaps lack shopworn, unsophisticated slogans and taglines as their appeal lies in unique ingredients, packaging, and scents.

What is causing this soap phenomenon? According to Faith Popcorn, a well-known trend forecaster, "Stressed-out consumers are on the lookout for affordable, small luxuries. They seek ways to reward themselves at an affordable level." Soap fits the bill.

A lot of entrepreneurs have therefore jumped on this burgeoning specialty soap market. There are even soap associations, soap-maker guild websites, and a soap makers' magazine, *Saponier*. Specialty soap makers have found markets for their products in all kinds of outlets, including bath and beauty stores, spas, natural food shops, and department stores. Many have opened their own shops.

In order to distinguish their unique products, they personalize, modify, and market in imaginative ways. Using their sensitive noses and discriminating eyes, they might throw in a little coconut, palm, olive, or sunflower oil, and infuse their concoctions with mixes of fragrant flowers, fruits, and even vegetables. Some stir in nuts and seeds to exfoliate the skin. Many add colors and even whimsical toy fish, ducks, and astronauts, to enhance the effect. Then they mold their soaps into attractive and frequently amusing shapes. Once an irresistible soap has been produced, many soap makers design eye-catching packaging for their products—Indonesian grass woven pouches, Victorian-era boxes tied with grosgrain ribbon, or exotic leaf wrappings from banana trees or cornstalks.

The minimalist white bar simply does not cut it for the specialty soap enthusiast. These customers are seeking a luxuriating, pampering, singular sensation. Soap can now be a collectible, a housewarming gift, or even a work of art.

Some soaps have even made a comeback, such as Dr. E. H. Bonner's soaps and cleansers, Peppermint 18-in-1 Pure-Castile soap, and the All-One. Created by a master chemist and rabbi, these weirdly packaged products have been a hit with hippies and hipsters since the 1960s. The products' unique labeling feature rambling, mini-manifestoes on topics such as overpopulation that read like stream-of-

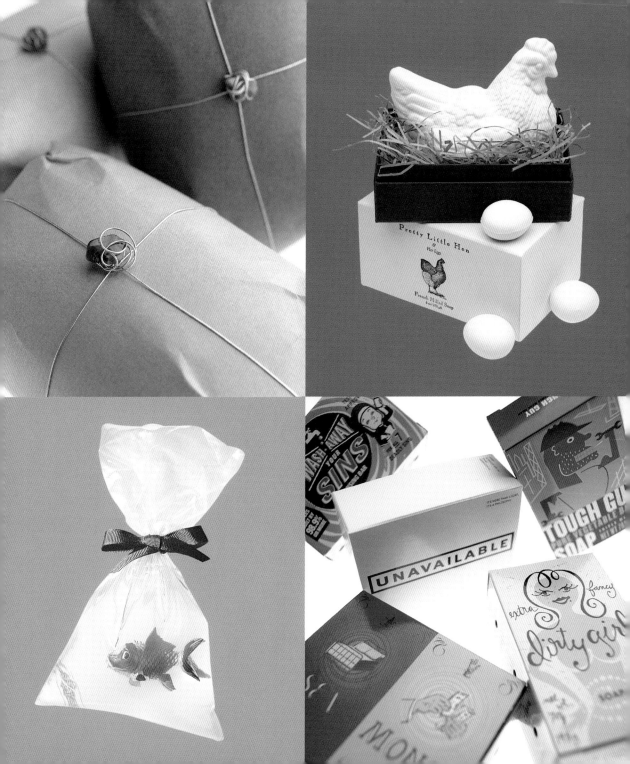

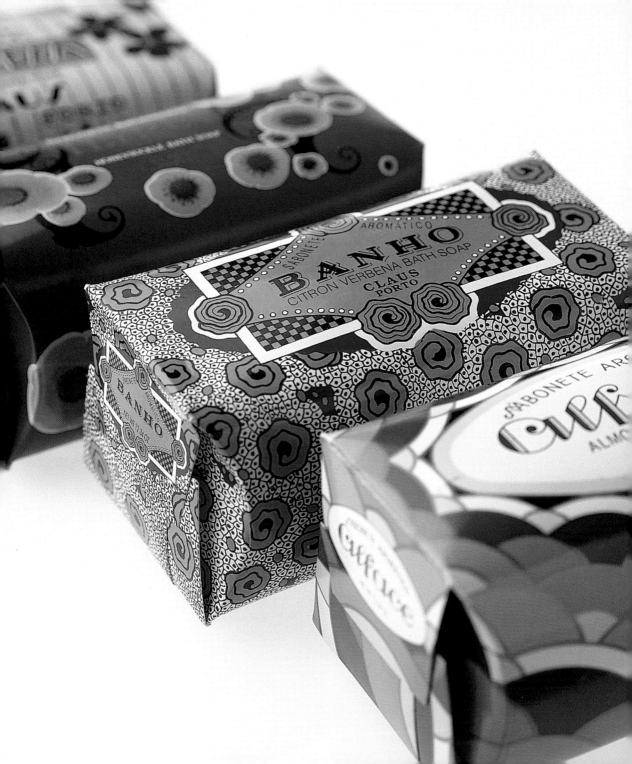

consciousness doggerel, and the soaps, now grossing over a million and half dollars a year, are sold mainly in health-food stores.

Simply Splashing, a South African company, is an example of a new soap brand coming into the market and succeeding. Included in this impressive line are Loofah soaps in which the exfoliating plant is submerged in glycerine. They come in six different essential oils. Other ingenious products are Soap Scrolls. Each of the nine-inch long soaps is rolled up like a crêpe and comes in one of a number of combinations, including redbush tea and honey; jasmine oil and poppy seed; neroli oil and sweet basil; and ylang ylang and rose petals.

Botanicals—especially fruit and vegetable soaps—are growing in popularity within the specialty soap niche. Ad copy makes them sound good enough to eat. Consider Fresh's pitch that its fruity line "has a bright and tart aroma which leave(s) your taste buds watering (and is) scented with the tangy zest of cranberry blended with the perfectly ripe essences of lemon, orange, cherry, or green apple."

Regardless of whether or not you can nourish your skin from the outside, you can still feel and smell great. Burt's Bees line of Complexion Soaps includes nourishing ingredients, such as Wild Lettuce (which contains dried lettuce leaves) or Garden Carrot (which boasts beta-carotene to cleanse pores). Fruits and spices are big, too. Emelauren's soaps, which are handcrafted in Pennsylvania, range from Glazed Apple with Pears and Plum to Spiced Cinnamon with Vanilla and Clove.

Lafco's Italian-made *Sapone per Cucina* offers six soaps containing tomato, eggplant, carrot, mango, fig, or pear fragrances. Jan Bresler, a former New York City lawyer who abandoned litigation for saponification, heads the company. In 1992, he traveled to Portugal, where he fell in love with Claus Porto's century-old soaps in Art Deco wrapping paper. Recognizing the boom ahead, Bresler began his own soap import company. Part of the firm's success lies in Bresler's aesthetic sensibility. "When I started, personal care was all brown paper, corrugated cardboard and raffia. Not very interesting," he remembers. "I wanted my company to be about home décor for the bathroom." His Kimono soaps from Japan are packaged in hand-screened Japanese Mingei papers and tied with a thick satin string.

Not to be outmarketed by increasingly competitive novelty, the T. S. Pink Corp. headquartered in Oneonta, New York, manufactures beautiful soaps which resemble rose quartz, amethyst, citrine, and malachite. "Each 'rock' is different. They are not mass-produced," says founder Todd Pink, a former geologist. "What we're making is fine art that is useful, smells wonderful, and that washes." Museum shops nationwide agree and are among the company's biggest retail outlets.

Imported from Japan, the Chidoriya line of soaps (established in 1949) takes a decidedly theatrical direction in their presentation. Originally made for Maiko dancing girls and geishas, the fashion and beauty trendsetters of Kyoto, the soaps' base is pure camellia and essential oils. These oils are all known for their ability to stimulate circulation, while helping the body release trapped accumulated toxins and fluids. Each soap is housed in an art deco pyramid.

In France, the Caudalie Company, created by Mathilde Cathiard Thomas and her husband, Bertrand, buys their soap ingredients from France's grape-producing provinces, including Champagne, Alsace, Provence, and Burgundy. The couple manufactures Ultra-Mild Wine soap. They found that the presence of antioxidants in red wine stabilizes grape seed polyphenols, which are believed to neutralize free radicals that cause skin wrinkles.

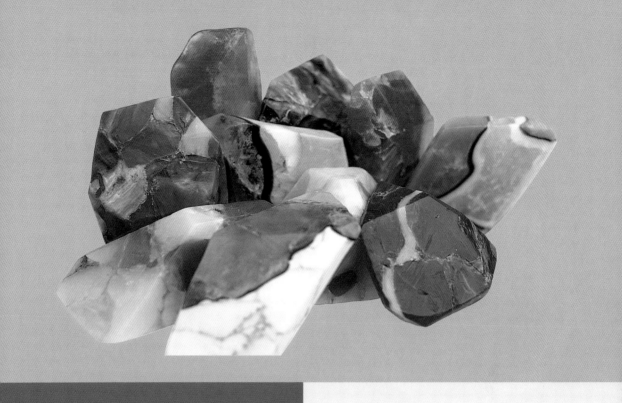

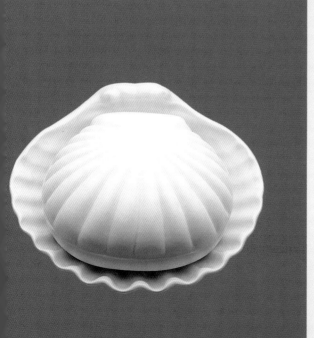

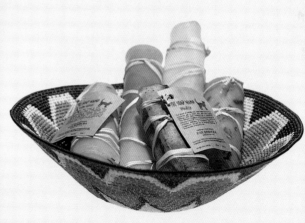

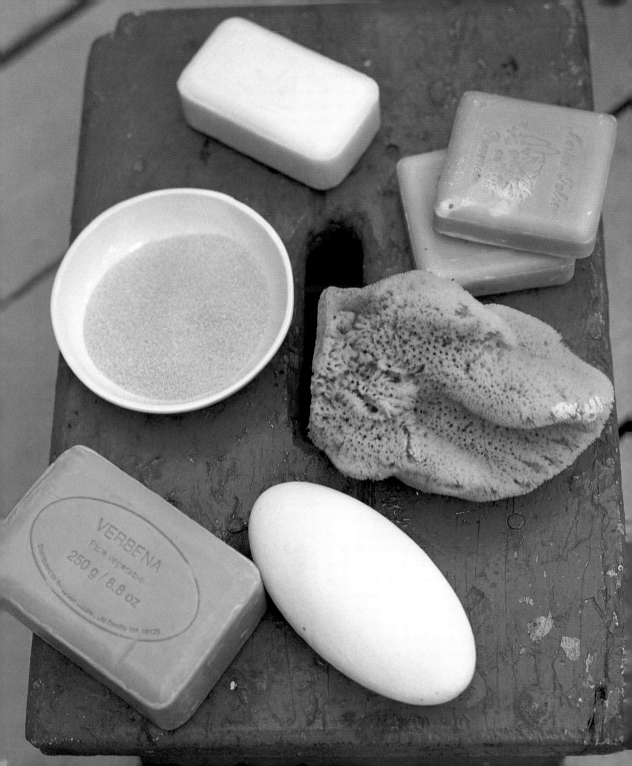

selecting the ideal soap

Soap selection is very subjective and very confusing. Antibacterial, superfatted, deodorant, triple-milled, glycerine, fragranced—every kind of soap is out there. Also available are bath salts and oils, liquid soaps, foaming shower gels, and more.

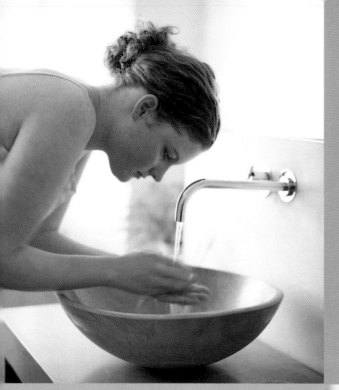

Clinique, one of the country's leading cosmetic firms, recommends a three-step washing system, especially for the face. First, cleanse with soap and water. Then exfoliate with a clarifying lotion. Finally, apply a moisturizer.

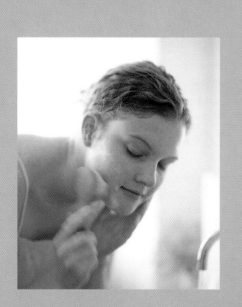

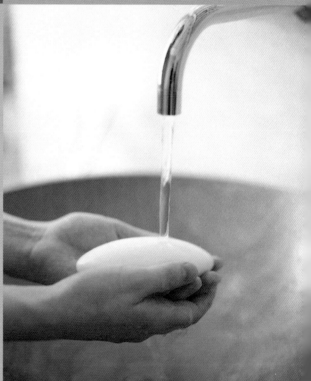

In order to select the perfect soap for yourself, a general understanding of your skin and your skin type is a must. Skin is the body's first line of defense. It is your protection against dirt and germs. It retains the body's fluids, protects us from the wind, water, and sun and it helps maintain the body's temperature through perspiration.

The *epidermis* (Greek for "upon the skin"), the outer layer of the skin, has at its base cells that are alive and growing. These growing cells push upward and away from the blood supply of the *dermis*, the second layer of our skin that we don't see. As these cells, thousands of them, move further away from the bloodstream they can no longer live and are constantly replaced with new cells.

The average person's combined epidermis and dermis adds up to about 7 percent of a person's total weight. Skin, which is about $\frac{1}{8}$-inch thick on the soles of the feet and much thinner on the face, measures about 20 square feet, weighs roughly nine pounds, and, quite astonishingly, is the largest organ of the human body.

Thousands of glands are distributed all over our dermis. It is through the pores at the end of these glands that healthy skin secretes sebum. Sebum is a waxy lipid mixture that reduces water loss from the skin surface and protects the skin from infection. If pores are blocked, this waxy lubricant results in blackheads. Pores on our foreheads and faces are more numerous and somewhat larger. This is why beads of perspiration can often be seen there before perspiration begins to appear elsewhere on our bodies. Our faces also have an elaborate network of sensory nerves, which is one reason one's face can become irritated so easily.

Odor occurs when there's a breakdown of organic substances caused by bacteria on our skin. Most people don't realize that it isn't the perspiration that causes body odor; it's the dead cells.

What this boils down to is that if left uncleansed, the skin becomes a breeding ground for germs. Regular cleansing protects our bodies from parasites. What soap does is that it washes away dead cells, removes organic substances deposited during perspiration, and carries off all the germs and dirt that has collected on us from our environment.

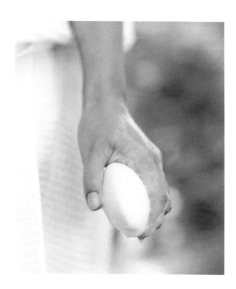

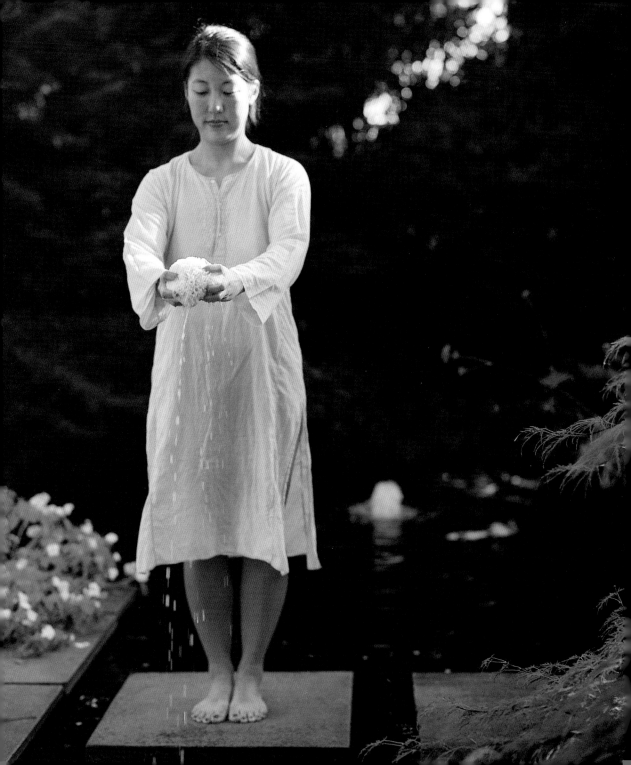

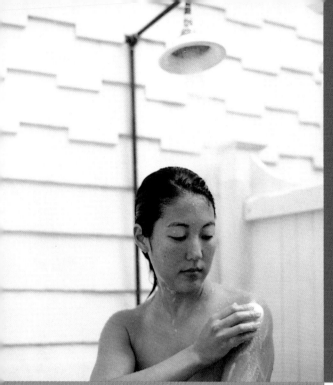

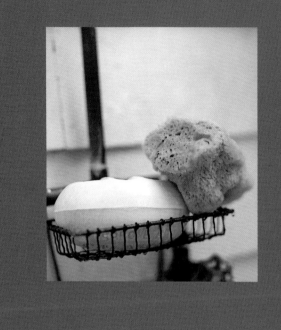

The right way to end a wash-up, according to the Erno Laszlo Skin Care Institute is, "Rinse, rinse, rinse." Clients are told to splash their faces at least thirty times after washing.

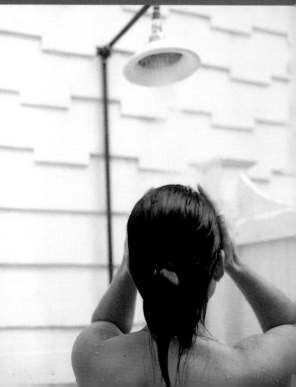

SOAP BASICS

Soaps are formulated today with the vast variety of human living conditions and subsequent skin needs in mind. Soap manufacturers are alert to climate conditions (cold and dry versus hot and muggy); the environment (especially city pollution); as well as the quality of water (hard versus soft).

Soap's cleansing power comes from its low surface tension. Soap, containing surfactants or wetting agents that allow oil and water to mix, breaks up the particles of dirt and oil. Surrounded by a film of soapsuds, which prevents them from again attaching to the surface being washed, the soil is suspended in the water, or emulsified, and by rinsing is washed away. In scientific terms, emulsion refers to the mixture of two mutually insoluble liquids in which one is dispersed in droplets into the other. In short, the oil and dirt on the surface of the skin are dispersed in the soap lather.

A common denominator among most soaps is the fact that they are milled. This is a process by which soap chips are thoroughly blended to ensure that additives and ingredients are evenly distributed, then compressed to remove moisture. If soap is triple-milled, it has been through the pressing process three times; therefore, practically no air remains. This makes triple-milled soap last longer; it also allows the addition of fine perfumes whose scents linger. The soap lathers better and is more moisturizing as well. And finally, because it doesn't absorb much water, triple-milled soap doesn't get as mushy and gloppy as some soaps do when they are left standing in water.

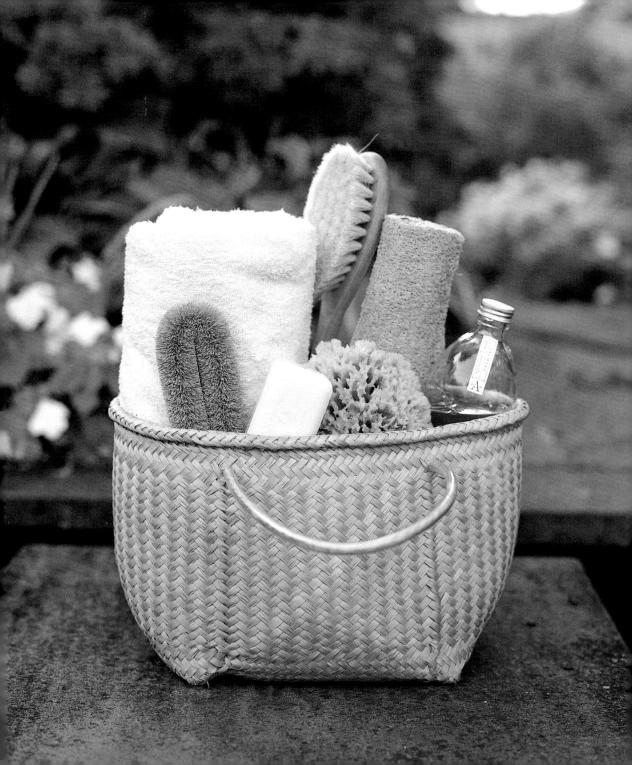

Everyone should evaluate his/her skin type. Keep in mind that yesterday's diagnosis may not be today's. Catherine Hinds, Director of the Catherine Hinds Institute of Esthetics, classifies the skin in seven different categories, which can often vary seasonally and which may overlap. Skin can be normal, oily, dry, a combination, mature, sensitive, and/or environmentally damaged. The ten top enemies to skin are: smoking, pollution, dry air, excessive pulling on the skin, abusive exfoliation and/or overzealous cleansing, alcohol, drugs, constipation, and ultraviolet rays.

The reason for a regular skin check-up, according to skin-care specialists, is that skin changes, usually after one is twenty-five years and older. Oil production slows down. And for women, skin reacts to hormonal changes during and after pregnancy and menopause. One should consult a good dermatologist regularly or even a licensed esthetician on the staff of a full-service salon or spa.

Before going any further, it should be pointed out that dermatologists and physicians now counsel against vigorous scrubbing with soap and water. Gentleness in skin care is the way to go. To have skin that is squeaky clean means that all the natural oils have been stripped off the skin surface. People with sensitive and/or oily skin should be particularly careful. Many soaps have a high alkaline content which can trigger glands into overdrive and cause them to pump out more oil. Using the wrong soap can also result in psoriasis, the dermatological name for chronic dry skin, which afflicts about a third of the population, especially older adults.

Gentle cleansing bars are increasingly popular. Since some soap manufacturers make cosmetic claims, the Food and Drug Administration requires that they list ingredients—a real plus according to Sandy Kuzmich, Ph.D., the Good Housekeeping Institute's chemistry director. "You need to know what's in a soap if you have dry skin," she says. According to specialists, if you have skin problems and want to use soap, be sure to select the very least alkaline soaps for your body that you can find. Remember as well, water is one of the best moisturizers. A ten to twenty minute bath is a great hydrator.

The way to judge if a soap is too strong (or alkaline) is to ask, "does my skin remain taut after being washed?" If your skin remains feeling stretched, switch soaps. Read soap labels to avoid soaps with a high (8 to 11) pH, which a majority of soaps do contain. Go for a gentler soap, one with emollients that seal in moisture and one which boasts a "balanced pH"; that is, one that closely matches the skin's usual acid level.

Even the mildest soap can dry out or irritate the skin if it isn't thoroughly rinsed off. "Because of its stripping action, soap can signal your glands to compensate by pumping out more oil," warns Carolyn Ash, a noted skin-care counselor in Dallas, Texas. This is especially true if the soap residue is trapped under a moisturizer. Residue from agents in soap can break down the skin's protective coat, thus causing dryness, even inflammation.

Caring for your skin should be a pleasant, invigorating experience. Enjoy all five senses while bathing by accessorizing your bathroom with aromatic soaps and candles, beautiful soap dishes, plush towels, and natural sponges, brushes, and pumice stones. Add some soothing music and a refreshing glass of water while you experience one of life's more relaxing moments.

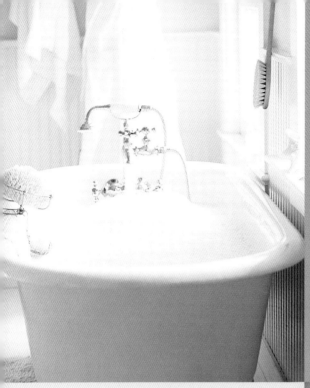

The bath is no longer a place just to get clean. To many, it has become a sanctuary: a place for relaxation and contemplation; a time to indulge yourself; an opportunity to cleanse your body and uplift your spirit.

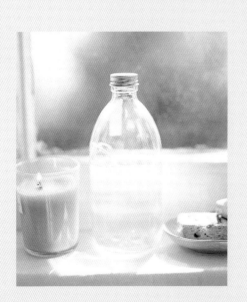

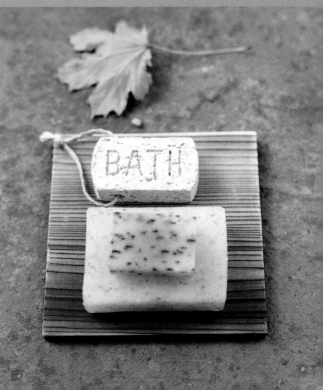

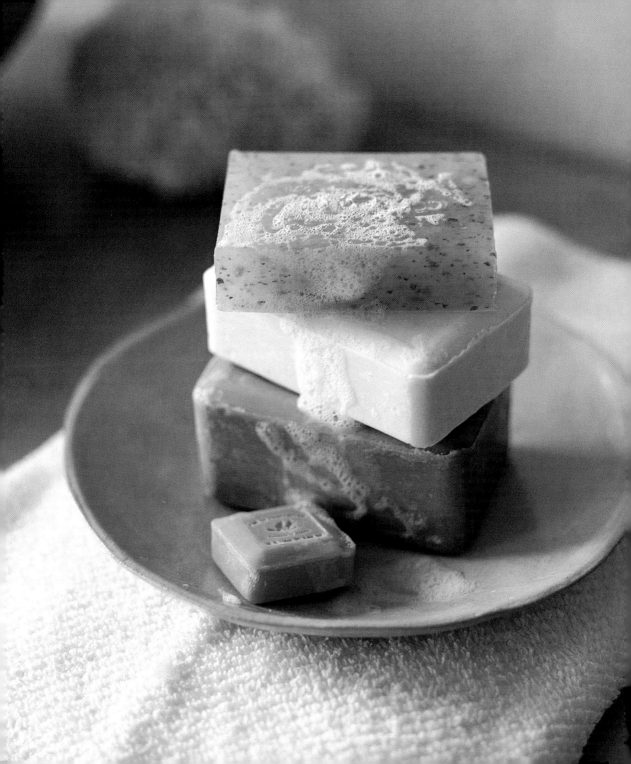

types of soap

When selecting soaps, you should read labels and find one that satisfies your particular skin requirement.

acne Low in oils and contains antiseptic ingredients that help to remove bacteria from the skin's surface. Washing two to three times a day is recommended to remove sebum and excess skin cells, which cause blockage.

antibacterial First used in hospitals, then introduced to the consumer market in 1994, antibacterial soaps make up more than 35 percent of all soaps sold nationwide in the United States. This is despite tests that show that while antibacterial soaps can be effective, they may also kill "friendly" bacteria, thus encouraging fungal infections.

castile Contain olive oil as their fat-base. They are excellent moisturizers.

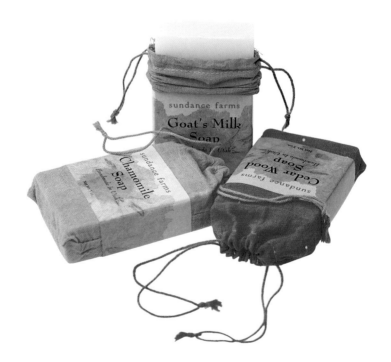

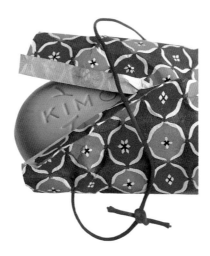

combar The word "combar" signifies a combination of soap and synthetic cleansers. Dove, Oil of Olay, Beauty Bar, and Whitewater Zest are among the leading brands. Beauty forecasters believe synthetic compounds in conjunction with the healing ingredients of certain botanicals are the wave of the future.

deodorant Contains antiseptics and sometimes perfume for controlling odor-causing bacteria. Because the key ingredients can irritate the face, it is best to use this kind of soap only on the body.

fragranced Fragrance, which serves as a preservative to keep soap sweet smelling and free from rancidity, can irritate sensitive and allergy-prone skin, especially the face. Therefore, it is best to use below the neckline. These soaps are wonderful for luxuriating in a bathtub, and can complement one's mood. Peppermint, rosemary, and juniper are said to enliven. Calendula and vanilla ease tension. And lavender relaxes.

french-milled Hard-milled, these soaps have minimal alkalinity and are good at oil removal.

glycerine With around a 10 percent glycerine level (versus regular soaps with only about ½ percent glycerine), these soaps are known for their smooth consistency and their transparency—although they may contain a bit of color. Their moisture-attracting properties are good for people with sensitive but oily skin. Since this kind of soap often contains both 80 proof vodka and whiskey, its production is monitored by the federal government in the United States.

hard-milled Ground down then compressed several times to make a dense, long-lasting soap.

superfatted Made with 5 to 15 percent fat (versus the 2 percent fat content of most soaps), this kind of soap contains a good deal of moisturizers, often lanolin. It is not known for its oil-removal.

synthetic (or detergent) According to Dr. Barney J. Kent, a dermatological surgeon at New York Presbyterian Hospital–Cornell Medical Center, "Even though the word 'detergent' might make you think of harsh laundry powder, in the world of skin care a synthetic detergent is often milder than soap. It also works well in whatever kind of water one is using, hard or soft." The pH of these soaps is ideal for dry and sensitive skin.

There are other factors to ponder as well. Consider all the different scents. There are dozens and dozens of them—herb and spice, fruit, vegetable, flower. Some favorites are grapefruit, mandarin, geranium, peppermint, balm mint, wintergreen, lavender, patchouli, marjoram, pine, bay, and bergamot. There are also different textures and fillers in soap, such as bran, almonds, herbs, seaweed, spices, wheatgerm, and pumice. Others contain additives such as avocado oil, aloe vera gel, milk, honey, and vitamin E oil.

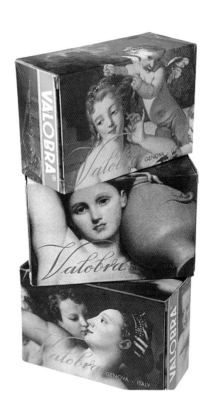

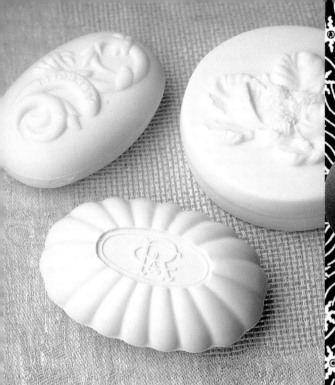
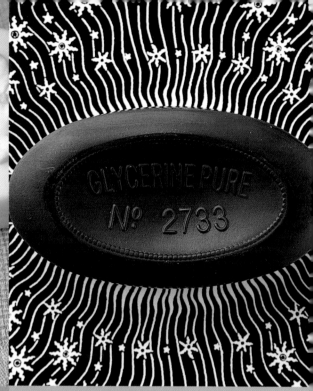
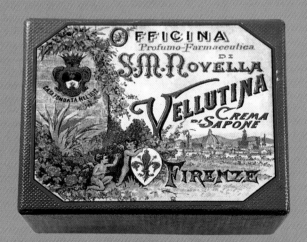
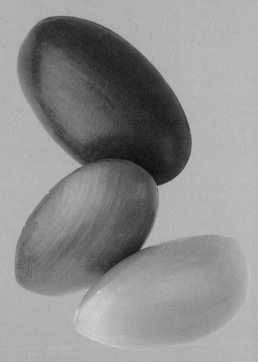

the soap marketplace

Now that you know what to look for in a soap, here is a brief overview of what some luxury soap companies have to offer. Remember, there are hundreds of soap companies around the world. The number grows daily. We regret we can only offer information on some of our favorites.

MAJA

In seventeenth-century Spain, the town of Castilla profited from the area's great groves of olive trees. Used exclusively by the town's soap-making companies, the local olive oil made the Castile soaps famous for their soothing feel to skin. Castile soap is now synonymous with olive oil soap made anywhere. Maja is probably Spain's best known soap brand, which is sold worldwide. Made with Spanish olive oil, Maja comes in a distinctive black-and-red wrapper that shows a beautiful señorita, or maja, fanning herself. Scented with rose, jasmine, and other flowers, the soap's formula is the same one perfected by the Myrurgia Company when it began business in Barcelona at the turn of the century.

L'OCCITANE EN PROVENCE

L'Occitane was founded by Olivier Baussan in 1976. He set out to capture Provence's most subtle fragrances and oils in his collection of bath, body, and hair products, and candles to delight the senses. L'Occitane, the ancient name for Provence, carries a large line of exceptional soaps ranging from mahogany-colored, forest-fragranced Linden Wood to 30 percent olive oil–based bars.

The company also offers exotic Shea Butter soaps made from moisturizing ingredients derived from the nut of the sacred shea tree of the West African country, Burkina Faso. Shea is known as "woman's gold," for according to tradition, only women are permitted to gather the nut. L'Occitane has developed a humanitarian partnership with these women to preserve the tradition. The soothing Shea Butter is used by African drummers to protect their fingers and hands.

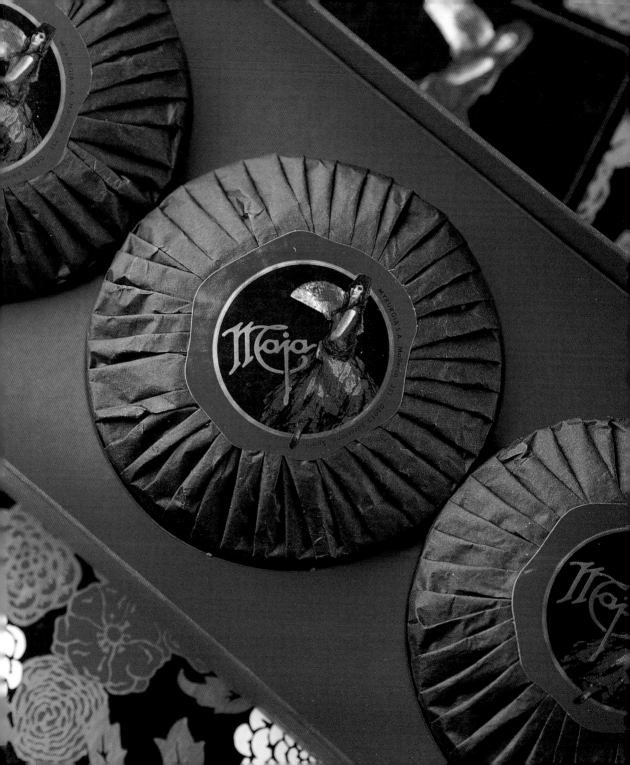

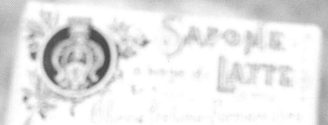

L'Occitane operates a museum of soap in Volx in Haute Provence called the Eco-Musée du Savon (open April through September). The collection features numerous vintage illustrations, photographs, and engravings of soap making during the last century, as well as antique bars of soap.

OFFICINA PROFUMO

L'Officina Profumo-Farmaceutica di Santa Maria Novella is said to be the oldest pharmacy in the world still doing business. Founded in Florence in 1612 by Dominican friars, the pharmacy's fame spread as far as Russia and China. Today, its main salesroom, a chapel built in 1335, is one of the city's—if not the world's—great visual and olfactory experiences. Passing through frescoed rooms full of furnishings and implements of a Renaissance pharmacist's trade, customers of all nationalities queue up to buy health and beauty products made from recipes perfected by the Brothers five centuries ago. Today Santa Maria Novella soaps—stamped and wrapped by hand—reflect this craftsmanship but use formulas that only date back to the 1850s. Still, many are made from the same medicinal plants and herbs the Brothers cultivated four centuries ago in the garden and are hand-molded and aged for sixty days. With outlets throughout Italy, and in London and Paris, L'Officina Profumo-Farmaceutica is noted for its *sapone al melograno*, pomegranate soap; *sapone alla mandorla*, almond soap; *sapone fior d'iris*, iris soap; and *sapone alla menta*, mint soap.

RANCE

Rancé is another well-known European soap company, which has been in business for centuries. During the late eighteenth century, the Rancé family was renowned for their glove making in Grasse, near Cannes in southern France. Their kid gloves were perfumed and sold primarily to the French aristocracy. After the French Revolution, François Rancé branched out and began a perfume factory. To Napoleon, he dedicated "The Winter's Perfume," to the Empress Josephine, "Empire."

In the late nineteenth century, Maison Rancé moved to Milan, Italy, where, seven generations later, the family continues to make perfume and scented soaps. The line of fine perfumed triple-milled soaps enriched with natural extracts and oils, as well as glycerine soaps are both sought worldwide.

ROGER & GALLET

Roger & Gallet, a French company headquartered in Paris, continues to make soap in an age-old fashion. An original recipe discovered by Armand Roger and Charles Gallet in 1695 (that was later updated) uses healing waters in the company's unique soap-making "cauldron-method." The recipes for the company's different soap lines are altered during this process to suit the needs of different skin types.

The basic ingredients for these soaps are oily acids and scrub soda, which are mixed for five hours. Next, the impurities are separated out by adding a salty solution, and the resulting mixture stands for as much as three hours. The soaps are further refined with three separate washings. Dried for forty-eight hours before being stored in wooden silos, the soaps are finally perfumed. Roger & Gallet soaps, wrapped in elegant pleated paper and packaged in colorful, plastic travel cases, are shipped to French pharmacies, as well as bath shops throughout the world.

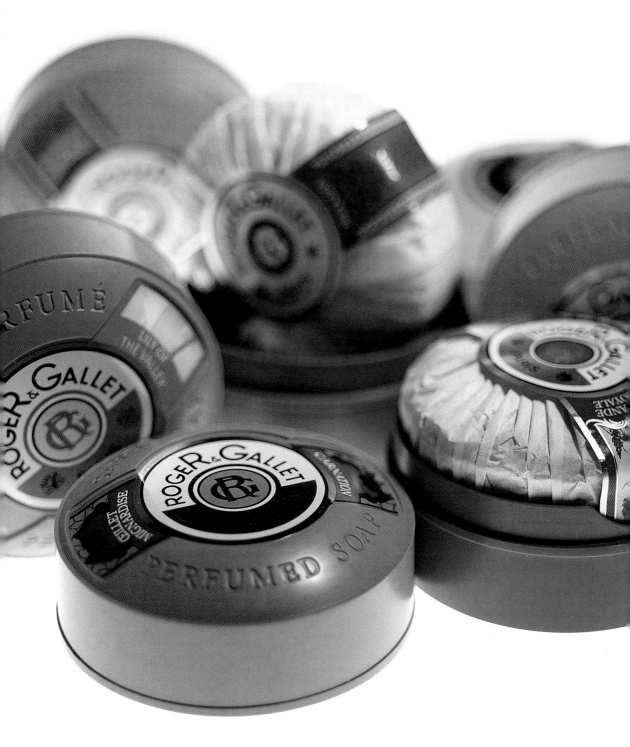

SAVONNERIE MARIUS FABRE

Savonnerie Marius Fabre in Salon de Marseilles in Provence, is one of the three remaining factories that maintains the historic manufacture of the world-famous *Savon de Marseilles*. Since the factory's inception, in 1900, the production of its multi-use soap has changed very little. To walk through the factory is to step into the past. Cauldrons bubble. Enormous troughs of soap "batter" are smoothed out with long-handled wooden spatulas. The air is rich with the fragrance of oil.

After employees have individually checked each cube of Fabre's *Savon de Marseilles* for defects, they cut the soaps by hand, then stamp each cube with its weight in grams. They also *"faire le marque,"* or stamp, each cube by hand with one of Fabre's many vintage insignias. Unscented and uncolored, the delicate, hypoallergenic soaps are beloved by bathers worldwide with sensitive skin. It is also a favorite laundry soap.

LA TOJA

According to folklore, a sick donkey was left to die on the island of La Toja off Galicia in northwestern Spain. Returning months later, the owner found the donkey alive and well. He attributed the animal's miraculous cure to therapeutic hot springs on the island. Eventually, La Toja became a spa.

Taking advantage of the local waters, the La Toja Company began production of its distinctive jet-black soaps in the early twentieth century, adding iron, iodine, and sulfur to its recipes in an effort to further the soaps' reputedly healthful benefits. Although a peculiar color for a vehicle of cleanliness, the black La Toja soaps nevertheless produce a thick white lather.

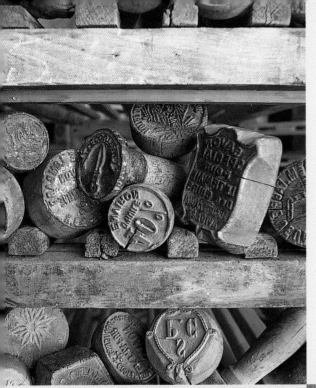
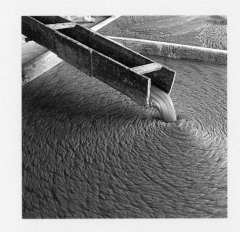
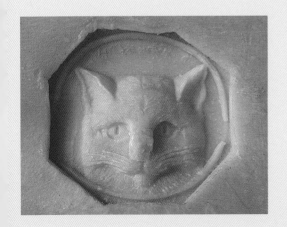
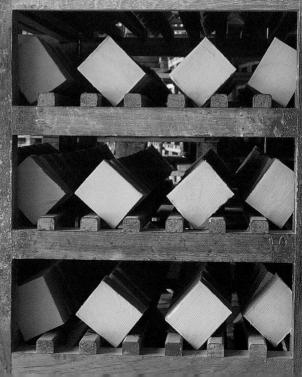

glossary of soap terms

The following are words commonly used in the soap industry, found on soap labels and on websites, and spoken by people passionate about soap.

Aromatherapy: The use and application to the body of natural, botanical, fragrant essential oils from flowers, resins, seeds, roots, bark, leaves, and plants. Each individual essence produces a specific beneficial effect to refresh, relax, or invigorate the user while inducing a soothing sense of well-being.

Baking Soda: A relaxing water softener, effervescent deodorizer, and a stimulant. Helps to draw oils and impurities from the skin.

Castor Oil: Oil extracted from castor oil beans in tropical Africa and Asia. Attracts and retains moisture to the skin; also serves as a thickener and emollient.

Cocoa Butter: Fat obtained from dried and naturally fermented cocoa beans cultivated primarily in Ghana, Ivory Coast, and Nigeria. Used in soap as a protector, moisturizer, skin softener, and emollient.

Coconut Oil: Oil from the fruit of the coconut palm grown in most tropical countries, including Sri Lanka, Mexico, India, Indonesia, and the Philippines. In soaps, it is an emollient that is protecting, conditioning, and moisturizing to the skin. It helps make a hard bar that produces a fast, sudsy lather.

Colorants: Either a natural or synthetic dye or pigment used to alter the color of a product. Names like "FD&C Blue" mean the colorant has government approval for use in foods, drugs, and cosmetics.

Detergent: Any of a group of synthetic, organic, liquid, or water-soluble cleaning agents that, unlike soap, are not prepared from fats and oil.

Emollient: Anything that has a softening effect on the skin.

Emulsion: A blending of two normally incompatible liquids in which one is dispersed in the other, including oil-in-water and water-in-oil emulsions.

Essential Oils: Pure extracts and distillates which make the smell associated with plant roots, resins, rinds, berries, stems, leaves, vegetables, and flowers.

Exfoliate: To cleanse away dead skin to remove deeply trapped secretions that impede oxygenation.

Glycerine: A colorless liquid extracted from vegetable fats. A by-product of soap making—glycerine is separated from fatty acids. It is an emollient and a humectant.

Humectant: An ingredient that promotes retention of moisture.

Jojoba Oil: Penetrating oil similar to natural human oil secretions. Excellent skin conditioner; especially for inflammations, acne, psoriasis, and eczema.

Loofah: Any of several tropical vines of the gourd family used to exfoliate the skin and stimulate circulation.

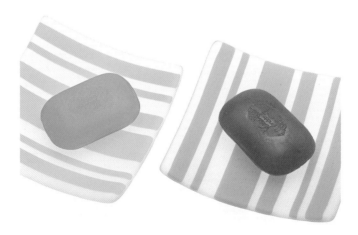

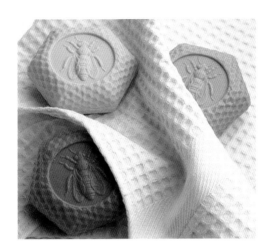

Lye: Caustic alkali used in soap making. Can refer to either potassium hydroxide (potash) or to sodium hydroxide (caustic soda).

Marbling: The effect achieved by mixing two different colored soaps together.

Olive Oil: Oil pressed from the fruit of olive trees grown primarily throughout the Mediterranean. Holds moisture close to the skin and therefore prevents loss of internal moisture. "Castile" soaps originally used only olive oil.

Palm Oil: Oil from the fruit of palm trees found mainly in Malaysia, Indonesia, and West Africa. Creates a hard bar of soap less soluble in water, which therefore retains firmness throughout use.

Pigments: Substances, frequently mineral, which add color to something else.

Potash: Originally derived by filtering water through hardwood ash. Also called potassium hydroxide, it is the caustic alkali in soft and liquid soaps.

Saponification: The reaction between the fatty acids in animal fat or vegetable oil and caustic alkali (lye) that produces soap.

Shea Butter: Also known as *karite* butter. A solid vegetable fat rendered from the nuts of a West African tree. Able to repair cellular degeneration, it has been used for centuries for treatment of skin disorders. Excellent for protection from sun and wind, to restore dry skin, and to treat blemishes, discoloration, scars, and wrinkles.

Sisal: A plant native to the tropics and used for its fiber as an exfoliating agent in soap.

Sodium Bicarbonate: Also known as baking soda. A soothing water softener; also deodorizing, effervescent, and stimulating. Draws impurities and oils from the skin.

Sodium Hydroxide: A caustic alkali used in hard soaps, which is made by processing salt water.

Superfatted: A soap composition containing 5 to 15 percent fat and a lot of moisturizers, such as lanolin.

Surfactant: Any substance that, when dissolved in water, reduces the surface tension or interfacial tension between it and another liquid.

Vitamin E: A good moisturizing oil. Also an antioxidant that helps protect cells from free radicals (high energy oxygen molecules absorbed from ultraviolet rays).

Wheat Germ Oil: Oil from the embryo of a wheat grain. Contains protein, minerals, and vitamins (especially vitamin E). An emollient, antioxidant, and natural preservative good for treatment of aged skin, eczema, and psoriasis.

resource guide

There are hundreds of soap makers, soap distributors, and soap stores all over the world. The number grows daily to satisfy the public's seemingly insatiable love of suds. The following is an abbreviated list of established soap companies, distributors, and stores that sell retail to customers. Remember, website addresses often change.

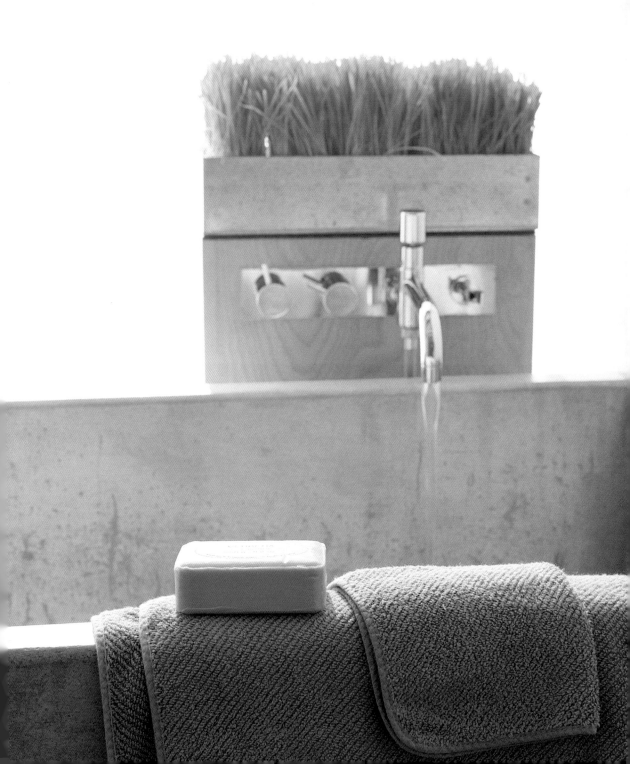

Amaranthine Aromatics

www.amaranthine.com

800.842.8609

Using essential oils and herbal ingredients, this botanically conscious company offers pH balanced aromatherapy soaps. Check out their Chandrika Ayurvedic line.

Barclay-Crocker

www.barclaycrocker.com

631.283.8012

This is a real find. A Southampton, New York, soap store with an informative and often humorous website detailing more than 100 bath, body, and home products. "Old guard" soaps share space with new arrivals.

Baudelaire

www.baudelairesoaps.com

800.327.2324

Importer of more than 100 international soaps, mainly from small, family-run European companies. Brands include: Provence Santé, Apiana, Jardin de l'Olivier, and Essence.

Bigelow Chemists

www.bigelowchemists.com

800.793.5433

The catalogue of this 160 year-old Greenwich Village apothecary is a treasure trove of personal care products. Soaps from Claus Porto in Portugal and Valobra in Italy are favorites.

Bliss

www.blissworld.com

888.243.8825

Bliss is the undisputed "hippest" spa in New York. The stylish website is complete with everything from tips on going to a spa to an online catalogue. Their body and skin-care products use the highest quality natural products.

The Body Shop

www.bodyshop.com

800.263.9746

Started in 1976 by Anita Roddick in England, The Body Shop is committed to environmental and social issues. The international company's vast line of natural bath and body products includes Vitamin E, Cocoa Butter Cream, and White Musk soaps.

Body Time

www.bodytime.com

888.649.2639

This cost-conscious California company offers biodegradable soaps, some with no fragrance or color additives, in two product lines: aromatherapy olive oil and glycerine.

Botanical Bath & Body Essentials

www.geocities.com/botanicalbath

614.294.2922

A botanical and natural line of pure, all-vegetable aromatherapeutic soaps, including Apple Jack, Bay Rum, Tangerine, Patchouli, and Ginger Lemongrass. The number is voicemail only, but they will call you back.

Bronnley of London Inc. – USA

www.bronnleyusa.com

800.383.1221

Established in 1883 in London, H. Bronnley & Co. Ltd. strived to become "makers of the best soap in the world." More than one-hundred years later, Bronnley holds three British Royal Warrants as suppliers to HM The Queen, HM Queen Elizabeth The Queen Mother, and HRH The Prince of Wales. Delectable suds result from

lathering up with Apricot and Almond, White Iris, and Blue Poppy, to name a few of the firm's extensive line. Custom blended soaps are made for notable department stores throughout the world. Bronnley of London Inc. – USA is a wholly owned company of H. Bronnley & Co. – UK.

Caswell-Massey

www.caswellmassey.com

866.227.9355

America's oldest chemist and perfumer, established in 1752, Caswell-Massey continues to make historic soaps, including its famous Number Six, a favorite of George Washington, as well as such classics as Almond Cold Cream and Cucumber.

Chianti Cashmere Company

www.chianticashmere.com

39.057.77.38.080

An expatriate American, Nora Kravis, herds more than one-hundred cashmere goats on seventeen acres in the breathtaking Tuscan valley of Radda in Chianti. Her cashmere goat farm produces natural goat-milk-based soaps, creams, and lotions, with no artificial additives or perfumes.

Crabtree & Evelyn

www.crabtree-evelyn.com

800.272.2873

A prime source of specialty soaps where one can buy luxurious triple-milled Avocado, Nantucket Briar, Lily of the Valley, and Chamomile soaps, as well as glycerine bars. This popular soap maker has retail stores worldwide.

Fresh

www.fresh.21c.com

212.396.0344

Fresh's creatively packaged products are known for their unique combination of natural ingredients and fragrances. The soaps are as beautiful as they are therapeutic.

French Soaps, Ltd.

www.frenchsoaps.com

888.511.7900

A wide range of French soaps made by legendary old-world *savonneries* includes Apothecaire, Esprit de Famille, and Doux.

Garden Botanika

www.gardenbotanika.com

800.968.7842

This company specializes in botanically and naturally based skin, hair, and body products. Their soaps are made of mud, sea kelp, and seaweed, among other ingredients.

Halcyonday Unlimited

www.halcyonday.com

800.350.9310

A wide selection of soaps from many worldwide companies, including Roger & Gallet, Kama Sutra, Terra Nova, and Davies Gate.

Juniper Imports

www.lifebuoy.co.uk

020.888.87360

This website carries two historic soaps: the original red Lifebuoy bar and Vinolia, a soap that A. & F. Pears Ltd. provided for the first class cabins of the Titanic, the ill-fated luxury liner.

Kiss My Face

www.kissmyface.com

800.262.KISS

Natural and organic, cruelty-free health and beauty products. With 86 percent olive oil content, soaps include Olive and Chamomile, Olive and Aloe, and Olive and Honey.

Lush

www.lush.co.uk

888.733.LUSH

Luxury bath melts, solid shampoos, loaf soaps and massage bars are among this super-trendy British company's vast soap offerings, available both online and in its many retail outlets. Products have wonderful names, such as Angels on Bare Skin and Dream Cream.

Maja Soap

www.majasoap.com

718.831.9313

Made in Spain, Maja soaps are exotically wrapped in pleated black paper. Customers worldwide lather up with Maja, Passion de España, or Embrujo de Sevilla.

L'Occitane en Provence

www.loccitane.com

888.623.2880

Throughout the year, annual verbena, lavender, and olive harvests produce limited-edition products to fit the season. Their soap specialties also include African shea butter soaps and wood-grained ergonomically designed soaps in linden, cedar, ebony, rosewood, and sandalwood, which are scented with tree roots and resins.

Penhaligon's

www.penhaligons.co.uk

877.736.4254

Established in 1870 in London, this perfumery's line of deliciously scented soaps includes several Royal Family favorites: Hammam, Lily of the Valley, English Fern, and Blenheim Bouquet.

Pharmacopia Botanicals

www.pharmacopia.net

877.389.9898

Using aromatherapy-grade essential oils for therapeutic qualities and exquisite aromas, the company's soaps are ribbed so they don't slip from one's hand. Try Serenity with lavender, Energy with rosemary and mint, and Bliss with ginger and lemongrass.

Pharmazie

www.luxbath.com

800.589.2284

A supermarket of more than fifty great soaps made by national and international companies. Categories include bar, bath, and homemade soaps.

T. S. Pink Corp.

www.tspink.com
800.762.7765
Todd Pink, a former geologist, is an "alchemist" whose ingenious Amber Citrine, Black Opal, and Rose Quartz SoapRocks are but a few faux bijoux in his dazzling collection of semiprecious soap creations. Each is a collector's item!

Officina Profumo-Farmaceutica di Santa Maria Novella

www.smnovella.com
39.055.84.89.873
Fax: 39.055.84.89.873
Begun in the seventeenth century by Dominicans, this landmark Florentine pharmacy tantalizes customers who come here from around the world to buy bath and beauty products from centuries-old recipes. Deliciously scented soaps include Potpourri, Pomegranate, and Mint. No web sales, only fax.

Savonnerie Marius Fabre

www.marius-fabre.fr
33.04.90.53.24.77
Fax: 33.04.90.53.41.54
Made from copra, palm, and olive oil, the soaps from this esteemed old-world company in southern France come in many shapes and sizes.

Scentier

www.scentier.com
888.522.6600
Represented here are scores of different companies' soaps, including those made by Essence, Provence Santé, La Compagnie de Provence, and Geo. F. Trumper.

Sephora

www.sephora.com
877.737.4672
Owned by the international conglomerate LVMH, the company sells Lady Bug, Piggy, and Rubber Duckie soaps from Bathology; Colloidal Oatmeal Health from Philosophy; and moisturizing, vegetable soaps from Erbe, plus more than 100 other brands.

Soap Box

www.soapboxltd.com
800.426.9260
In business twenty-six years, the company imports hundreds of the finest European soaps, including Pré de Provence, Via Borghese, and Oliviers & Co.

Soap on a Rope

www.soaponarope.com
888.773.7295
This website has everything from the classic soap with a rope attachment to a novelty medieval line, which is popular with Hollywood. The adorable children's line includes soap teddy bears and pets.

Soap Opera

www.thesoapopera.com
800.251.7627
A supplier of fine body-care products including world-famous Pears' glycerine soap with fragrances of cedar and rosemary. Also featured are hand-cut soaps in more than fifty fragrances and designs.

The Soap Shop

www.thesoapshop.com
207.967.8336
The company offers an extensive line of soaps, many hard to find and from abroad. Roger & Gallet soaps are scented with vetiver, magnolia, and fern. Lafco's line smells of wild pansy, red poppy, and almond.

Sunfeather Natural Soap Company

www.sunsoap.com
315.265.3648
Offers fine handmade soaps, soapmaking books, supplies, and equipment. A percentage of the proceeds from the sale of certain soaps go to various charities, for example, Washy Squashy children's soaps go to Stop It Now.

The Thymes

www.thymes.com
800.366.4071
Eucalyptus Glycerine, Fig Leaf and Cassis, and Green Tea are among the deliciously scented soaps in the company's large line of bath and body products.

Woodspirits Ltd.

www.woodspirits.com
937.663.4327
Biodegradable, minimally packaged soaps in recycled papers. Zanzibar, Salad Bar, and Phome are among this company's all-natural loaf soaps.

contributors

DESIGN AND ART DIRECTION: Nina Barnett
EDITORS: Sandra Gilbert and Elaine Schiebel
PRODUCTION MANAGER: Pamela Schechter

Product Shot Photography

PHOTOGRAPHER: Lisl Dennis
PHOTOGRAPHY ASSISTANT: Wendy McEahern
pages 6 (left to right) Mandarine, Soku Lime, Teak, Rain (Votivo Ltd., Seattle, WA); 7 (upper right) Bouquet Imperial (Roger & Gallet, Paris, France); 8 various *Savon de Marseilles* soaps; 14 (bottom right) *savon-beldi*, black olive-based soap, in a Moroccan *hammam*; 17 *Savon de Marseilles* bar soaps at the market in Isle sur la Sorgue, France; 28 (clockwise) Cocoa, Zea, Apricot Rose, Azena (Moonflower, Ranchos de Taos, NM); 31 (upper left/clockwise) Wisteria, Hesperides, Verbena (Fresh, Boston, MA); (upper right) Pretty Little Hen (Gianna Rose Atelier, Fountain Valley, CA); (bottom right/clockwise) Wash-Away Your Sins, Unavailable, Tough Guy, Dirty Girl, Sex/Money (Blue Q, Pittsfield, MA); (bottom left) Pet Fish glycerine soap (Bathology, Oakland, CA); 32 (front to back) Almond Oil, Citron Verbena, Honeysuckle, Wild Pansy, (Lafco, NY/Claus Porto, Portugal); 35 (top/clockwise) opal, turquoise, malachite, jasper, marble, lapis lazuli, rose amethyst, smoky quartz, amethyst (SoapRocks, T. S. Pink Corp., Oneonta, NY); (bottom right) African Healing Marula Soap Wand, (Pax Bodicea, South Africa/distributed by Shades of Africa, Jersey City, NJ); (bottom left) Savon Coquillage (Crabtree & Evelyn, Woodstock, CT); 50 (clockwise) Goat's Milk, Cedar Wood, Chamomile (Sundance Farms, Charleston, UT); 51 Lavender Kimono Soap, (Lafco, NY); 53 (top to bottom) Sapone Finissimo Lavana, Sapone Finissimo Fougere, Sapone Finissimo Rosa (Virgilio Valobra, Genoa, Italy); 54 (upper left/clockwise) Bronnley Classic Soap (London, England), Place de Lice Refreshing Soap (Milan, Italy), and Maison Rancé Crème Savon Extra Fine (Milan, Italy); (upper right) Glycerine Pure No. 2733 (Jabón Suavidad/imported by the Kala Corp., East Greenwich, RI); (bottom right) Savon Bois de Senteur (L'Occitane, Provence, France); (bottom left) Crema Sapone (Officina Profumo-

Farmaceutica di Santa Maria Novella, Florence, Italy); 57 Maja (Myrurgia S. A., Barcelona, Spain); 61 Perfumed soaps (Roger & Gallet, Paris, France); 63 details from Savonnerie Marius Fabre (clockwise) antique soap stamps, soap "batter" poured into troughs, drying racks, *Le Chat* (the cat) logo for one of the oldest brands of *Savon de Marseilles*; 67 Glycerine soaps (Fragonard, Grasse, France); 68 (clockwise) Honey, Gardener, and Propolis, Apiana Honeycomb soaps (Baudelaire, Keene, NH).

Lifestyle Photography

PHOTOGRAPHER: Ericka McConnell
PHOTOGRAPHY ASSISTANTS: Clare Chong and E. Celeste Marshall
MODELS: Claire Raibourn and Erin Shigaki
STYLIST: Loren Simons
front and back cover, title page, pages 7 (upper left and bottom right), 10, 13, 14 (upper left and right), 18, 22, 25, 36, 38, 40, 41, 42, 44, 47, 48, 58, 64, 71, 80.

Locations

Christina and Joseph Reddings' home in Southampton, New York: pages 7 (bottom right), 10, 18, 22, 36, 40, 41, 42, 44, 47, 58, 64, 80.
Patrick Orban's Soho loft, New York City: front and back cover, title page, pages 7 (upper left), 13, 14 (upper left and right) 25, 38, 48, 71.

Soaps and Accessories

The following items are available from the stores listed below.
Courtesy of Ad Hoc, New York: pages 25 (bottom right) Medallion soap, 48 Acca Kappa milk soap.
Courtesy of La Cafetière, New York: page 64 Italian horn oval soap dish.
Courtesy of Takashimaya New York: pages 7 (upper left) natural sea sponge, Fragonard Parfumeur soap, 14 (upper right) Blanc Savon, 25 (upper right) natural sea sponge, Côté Bastide soap.

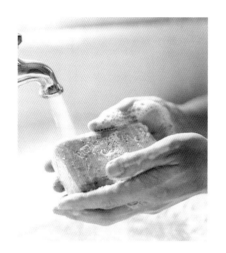

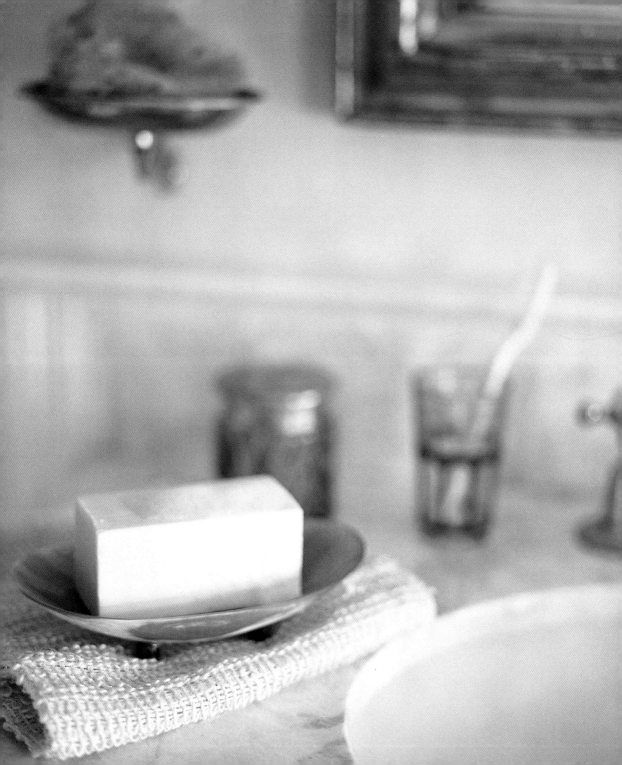